ESSENTIAL GUIDE TO SQUAMOUS CELL CARCINOMA

Understanding, Managing, and Conquering Squamous Cell Carcinoma: An In-Depth Guide for Patients and Caregivers

DR. CASEY LOREN

© 2024 by CASEY LOREN

All rights reserved .Except for brief quotations included in critical reviews and certain other noncommercial uses allowed by copyright law, no part of this book may be reproduced, distributed, or transmitted in any form or by any means, including photocopying, recording, or other electronic or mechanical methods, without the publisher's prior written permission.

DISCLAIMER

This book's content is only meant to be used for general informative purposes. Although the author has taken great care to ensure the content is accurate and thorough, no warranties or assurances on the information's accuracy, correctness, or reliability are provided. It is recommended that readers employ their own judgment and discretion when applying any material found in this book to their particular situation.

The information in this book is not intended to replace professional advice, nor is the author an expert in any of the subjects covered. It is recommended that readers consult with experienced professionals regarding any particular issues or concerns.

Any name that may be mentioned or referred in this book does not imply endorsement, recommendation, or relationship on the part of the author with any person, entity, good, website, or association. These references are made only for informational purposes and are not meant to be taken as recommendations or endorsements.

The information contained in this book may cause readers to suffer loss or damage, for which the author disclaims all obligation and accountability. The only people accountable for the decisions and actions taken by readers using the information presented are themselves.

Any names, characters, companies, locations, activities, occasions, and incidents referenced in this book are either made up or the result of the author's imagination. Any likeness to real people, living or dead, or to real things is entirely coincidental.

This book's content may change at any time, without prior notice, according to the author. The onus is on the reader to verify whether there have been any updates or revisions.

The reader accepts the conditions of this disclaimer by reading this book. Please do not read this book or use its contents if you do not agree to these terms.

Table of Contents

CHAPTER 1 16

SQUAMOUS CELL CARCINOMA: A COMPREHENSIVE OVERVIEW 16

Classification and Definition 16

Studies on the Causes and Prevention..........16

Squamous Cell Carcinoma Pathogenesis......17

Squamous Cell Carcinoma" Instances 17

Typical Venues and Demonstrations............18

Analytical Methods 18

Factors that indicate prognosis and stage 19

Diagnosis Varieties...19

Why Early Detection is Crucial.....................19

Recent Developments in the Rates of Incidence and Survival 20

CHAPTER 2 22

MOLECULAR AND CELLULAR PROCESSES 22

Origins in Cells and Histopathology 22

Changes at the molecular and genetic levels: 23

The Routes of Signal Transmission 23

The immune system's inner workings 24

Diagnostic Tools and Biomarkers: 24

Therapeutics with a Focus: 25

Methods for Immunotherapy 25

Epigenetics' Function: 26

Interactions between the Tumour Microenvironmen 26

New Areas of Study 27

CHAPTER 3 28

SIGNS AND SYMPTOMS IN THE CLINIC .28

Skin Problems and Their Morphology 28

Mucosal Lesions and Involvement of the Oral Cavity 29

Signs Seen by the Eyes...................................29

The Role of the Respiratory Tract 30

Symptoms in the Digestive System 30

Asymptomatic Genitourinary System...........31

Problems with the Nervous System 32

Neuroendocrine Disorders...........................32

Effects on Well-Being 33

Identifying SKUs and Kinds 33

CHAPTER 4...36

ANALYSIS OF HEALTH STATUS 36

Health History and Physical Assessment.....36

Methods for Conducting Biopsies and Analysing Their Results...............................37

Radiological Imaging Techniques (X-ray, CT, MRI, PET-CT): 37

Evaluation via Endoscopy: 38

Investigations Conducted in a Lab (Weapons Analysis, Cancer Detectors) 38

Genetic Analysis (NGS, PCR) 39

The Function of Liquid Biopsies: 39

Standards for Radiological Staging.............39

Diagnosis Through a Multidisciplinary Approach 40

Diagnostic Obstacles and Difficulties 40

CHAPTER 5 42

APPROACHES TO TREATMENT 42

Analysis of Margin and Resection Techniques in Surgery..42

Techniques and Targeted Approaches in Radiation Therapy.......................................43

Systemic treatments include molecularly targeted agents and chemotherapy 43

Immunotherapy New Approaches and Checkpoint Inhibitors..................................44

Thermodynamic Phototherapy 44

Electrochemotherapy is a treatment method. 45

Therapies Used in Combination...................45

Management of Symptoms and Palliative Care 46

Medicine as a Whole and Supplemental Treatments..46

Studies in Clinical Practice and Looking Ahead 47

CHAPTER 6..48

METHODS OF MANAGEMENT ORGAN SITE-BY-SITE..48

Squamous Cell Carcinoma of the Skin (CSCC) 48

Novel Squamous Cell Carcinoma of the Head and Neck (HNSCC)..49

Carcinoma of the Oesophagus......................50

Carcinoma of the Lung Squamous Cells 50

Carcinoma of the Cervical Squamous Cell....51

Cancer of the Anal Squamous Cell Line........51

The Cancer of the Genital Squamous Cells ..52

One Kind of Oral Cancer OSCC 52

Carcinoma of the Conjunctiva 53

Sites Uncommon and Uncommon Presentations 53

CHAPTER 7 56
MONITORING AND FOLLOW-UP TREATMENT 56

Protocols for Post-Treatment Monitoring ... 56

Monitoring Biomarkers 57

Counselling and psychological support: 57

Ongoing Management of Long-Term Effects and Complications 59

The Role of Lifestyle Changes 59

CHAPTER 8 62
TAKING PRECAUTIONS AND MINIMISING DANGER 62

Ways to Prevent Sun Damage 62

Programmes to Help People Quit Smoking . 63

Methods for Vaccination (e.g., Human papillomavirus) 64

Precautions for the Workplace 64

Suggestions for Food and Nutrition 65

Anti-Chemical Measures 65

Campaigns for Early Detection 66

Mitigating Environmental Risk Factors 67

Screening and Genetic Counselling 68

Programmes and Policies for Public Health 68

CHAPTER 9 70

ADVOCACY AND THE VIEWS OF PATIENTS 70

Stories of Patients' Journeys 70

Groups and Resources to Help 71

Groups that Speak Out for Causes 71

Programmes for Peer Mentorship 72

Resilience and Coping Mechanisms 73

Effects on Friends, Family, and Carers 73

Taking Care of People's Mental and Emotional Health 74

Aptitude for Health Information Exchange and Literacy 75

Encouraging Patients to Take Part in Decision-Making 76

Helping More People Have Access to Health Care 76

CHAPTER 10 78

A GLOBAL VIEW AND A LOOK AHEAD 78

The Worldwide Impact of Squamous Cell Carcinoma 78

Variations in Morbidity and Prognosis 78

Collaborations and Research on a Global Scale 79

New Approaches to Healthcare Delivery and Technology 80

Economic Analysis of Health Care and Interventions with Minimal Cost 80

Personalized Treatments and Precision Medicine 81

Problems with Putting Best Practices into Action 81

Healthcare Models Focused on Patients 82

Concerns Regarding Ethics in Cancer Care .82

Positive Movements and Encouragement ...83

CHAPTER 1

SQUAMOUS CELL CARCINOMA: A COMPREHENSIVE OVERVIEW

Classification and Definition

The outer layer of the skin contains flat cells called squamous cells, which can evolve into a form of skin cancer called squamous cell carcinoma (SCC). This skin cancer is among the most prevalent forms of skin cancer globally and is considered a non-melanoma.

Studies on the Causes and Prevention

Those over the age of 50 are more likely to develop SCC. But it's not limited to a certain age group. Prolonged sun exposure, a history of sunburns, pale skin, tanning bed use, radiation, a compromised immune system, specific chemical exposure, and a personal or family history of skin cancer are the primary risk factors for Squamous cell carcinoma (SCC).

Squamous Cell Carcinoma Pathogenesis

Sun exposure, both natural and artificial, including tanning beds, is the main risk factor for SCC development. Skin cells can develop malignant tumors when ultraviolet light destroys their DNA and causes mutations that cause squamous cells to expand uncontrollably.

Squamous Cell Carcinoma" Instances

Based on their outward manifestations and regional distribution, SCC subtypes can be distinguished. There are three types of SCC: cutaneous, mucosal, and metastatic. Cutaneous SCC affects the skin, whereas mucosal SCC affects the mucous membranes of organs like the throat, mouth, and genitalia.

Typical Venues and Demonstrations

Sun-exposed skin, including the face, ears, neck, scalp, hands, and arms, is a frequent site for SCC to develop. The most common symptoms include the development of a red, solid nodule or a scaly, ulcerating, bleeding patch. Constant sores, white spots, or a change in voice are all possible indications of mucosal SCC.

Analytical Methods

A skin biopsy is commonly used to confirm the presence of malignant cells during the diagnostic process of SCC, which also includes a comprehensive clinical evaluation. When metastasis is suspected, imaging tests such as MRI or CT scans may be ordered to determine the full extent of the disease.

Factors that indicate prognosis and stage

When deciding how to treat SCC, staging is a useful tool for gauging the extent of the cancer. Tumor size, lymph node involvement in the immediate area, and the occurrence of metastases to other parts of the body are common factors in this determination. The prognostic factors that impact treatment outcomes include the thickness and location of the tumor, as well as the patient's general health.

Diagnosis Varieties

Skin cancers such as SCC should be distinguished from benign skin lesions, basal cell carcinoma, melanoma, keratoacanthoma, and actinic keratosis. To make a correct diagnosis and choose the right treatment, this separation is vital.

Why Early Detection is Crucial

If SCC is detected early, treatment outcomes and prognosis will be much improved. To aid in early diagnosis and quick action, it is recommended to do regular skin inspections, self-check for changes in moles or skin lesions, and prompt medical evaluation of suspected lesions.

Recent Developments in the Rates of Incidence and Survival

Rising sun exposure, an aging population, and better detection methods are all factors in the recent uptick in SCC cases. Improved survival rates for people with SCC, especially when discovered early, have been achieved thanks to breakthroughs in treatment options including surgery, radiation therapy, immunotherapy, and targeted therapy.

To improve outcomes for patients with squamous cell carcinoma, healthcare providers and individuals must understand these features of SCC so that they can recognize the risk factors, symptoms, and indicators.

CHAPTER 2

MOLECULAR AND CELLULAR PROCESSES

Origins in Cells and Histopathology

The squamous cells that line the epithelium of several organs, including the skin, lungs, esophagus, and cervix, are the usual suspects in the development of squamous cell carcinoma (SCC).

- Pearl-like formations formed by atypical squamous cells with keratinization are histopathologically characterized by SCC. Differentiation levels in SCC can range from very high to very low.

To confirm that the tumor cells originate from the squamous cell line, immunohistochemical markers such as cytokeratins (e.g., CK5/6, CK7) are utilized.

Changes at the molecular and genetic levels:

Unchecked cell proliferation and tumor advancement are caused by genetic abnormalities seen in SCC, including mutations in TP53, NOTCH1, and CDKN2A.

Common molecular abnormalities in SCC, including as EGFR amplification and modifications to the PI3K-AKT-mTOR signaling pathway, affect cell survival and proliferation.

The Routes of Signal Transmission

In SCC pathogenesis, signaling pathways such as EGFR, MAPK, and Wnt/β-catenin are dysregulated, which leads to cell proliferation, invasion, and metastasis.

Activation of these pathways, it is worth noting, can cause resistance to traditional treatments.

The immune system's inner workings

Interactions among tumor cells, immune cells (such as T cells and macrophages), and cytokines make up the intricate immunological microenvironment of SCC.

-Inhibiting T cell activity and promoting tumor survival can be achieved through immune evasion mechanisms, such as the expression of PD-L1 on tumor cells.

Diagnostic Tools and Biomarkers:

- Genetic mutations, HPV status (in head and neck SCC), and PD-L1 expression are biomarkers that help in SCC diagnosis, prognosis, and therapy options.

Molecular diagnostic tools like next-generation sequencing (NGS) aid in the discovery of therapeutically relevant mutations.

Therapeutics with a Focus:

- Cetuximab is one example of an EGFR inhibitor; everolimus is a mTOR inhibitor; palbociclib is a CDK4/6 inhibitor; and there are many other targeted therapy for SCC.

By focusing on the chemical changes that fuel SCC formation, these treatments hope to reduce the likelihood of side effects.

Methods for Immunotherapy

To treat advanced SCC, immunotherapies that boost anti-tumor immune responses, such as immune checkpoint inhibitors (e.g., pembrolizumab, nivolumab), have proven to be effective.

To enhance the effectiveness of treatment, researchers are investigating the possibility of using immunomodulators in combination with targeted medicines.

Epigenetics' Function:

Epigenetic alterations, which regulate gene expression, have a function in the formation and progression of SCC. These modifications include DNA methylation and histone acetylation.

- One promising approach to treating SCC is to target epigenetic regulators, such as HDAC inhibitors and DNA methyltransferase inhibitors.

Interactions between the Tumour Microenvironmen

Squamous cell carcinoma (SCC) development, invasion, and therapeutic response are impacted by tumor microenvironmental interactions including tumor cells, stromal cells, and extracellular matrix components.

- Investigations are underway into strategies that aim to target the tumor microenvironment, such as stromal targeting treatments and anti-angiogenic medicines.

New Areas of Study

Personalized treatment approaches for SCC, better understanding the causes of therapy resistance, and discovering new therapeutic targets are the current areas of attention in the field of research.

Research and clinical management of SCC will be shaped in the future by advances in computational modeling, liquid biopsies, and single-cell sequencing.

Highlighting the multifaceted character of squamous cell carcinoma's cellular and molecular pathways, this thorough guide covers both the basic features and recent advances in the field.

CHAPTER 3

SIGNS AND SYMPTOMS IN THE CLINIC

Skin Problems and Their Morphology

On sun-exposed parts of the body such as the ears, neck, scalp, hands, and face, squamous cell carcinoma skin lesions might seem like red, crusty, or scaly patches. These sores have the potential to worsen with time, eventually becoming solid, elevated, and occasionally ulcerated with a crater in the middle. Their color ranges from pink to red to brown, and they can look like warts or sores that don't heal. A keratotic or horn-like appearance can be observed in certain SCC lesions. It's important to keep an eye on skin lesions and get them checked out if they change in size, form, or color. If they seem suspicious or if they continue, it's best to consult a doctor.

Mucosal Lesions and Involvement of the Oral Cavity

Mucosal surfaces, including those of the mouth and throat, are not immune to squamous cell carcinoma. Lesions can manifest as non-healing lumps, ulcers, or areas of white or redness. They may manifest in the oral cavity, gums, inside of the cheeks, palate, or neck. Some of the symptoms that may be experienced include discomfort, trouble swallowing, changes in flavor, or ongoing muscle aches. For the early diagnosis and treatment of mucosal lesions associated with SCC, it is vital to have regular dental exams and oral cancer screenings.

Signs Seen by the Eyes

The conjunctiva, a delicate and transparent membrane that covers the white portion of the eye and inner eyelids, can be affected by squamous cell carcinoma in extremely rare instances. A growth or mass on the surface of the eye can be an indicator of ocular SCC, which can lead to redness, swelling, tears, and alterations in vision. To diagnose and treat ocular symptoms of SCC promptly, it is crucial to consider a patient's visual acuity.

The Role of the Respiratory Tract

Lungs and airways are potential sites of SCC development. A chronic cough, difficulty breathing, chest discomfort, blood in the mucus, wheezing, or frequent respiratory infections are all possible symptoms. To assess respiratory involvement and direct treatment decisions—which may include a multidisciplinary approach involving pulmonologists, oncologists, and thoracic surgeons—imaging techniques, such as chest X-rays or CT scans, are crucial.

Symptoms in the Digestive System

Although it is uncommon, squamous cell carcinoma can develop in the mouth and throat, namely in the anal canal and esophagus. Discomfort when swallowing (dysphagia), chest discomfort, decreased appetite, and vomiting are all symptoms of esophageal squamous cell carcinoma (SCC). A mass around the anus, changes in bowel habits, bleeding, or anal pain could be symptoms of anal SCC. To diagnose and stage gastrointestinal SCC, diagnostic imaging, biopsies, and endoscopic procedures are required.

Asymptomatic Genitourinary System

Germinal and urinary tract organs including the cervix, penis, vulva, vagina, bladder, and urethra are all potential sites for SCC to grow. Urinary symptoms like pain or blood in the urine, changes in urinary habits, irregular vaginal bleeding, and genital ulcers are all possible outcomes of genitourinary SCC. Imaging investigations, gynecological exams, and urological evaluations can contribute to the diagnosis and management of genitourinary SCC.

Problems with the Nervous System

When squamous cell carcinoma progresses to an advanced stage, it poses a threat to the nervous system by metastasizing to nerve cells. Headaches, convulsions, limb weakness or numbness, altered mental status, and language difficulties are all possible symptoms. To diagnose and treat neurological disorders connected to SCC, one must undergo neurological evaluations, imaging tests (such as MRI), and consult with neurosurgeons.

Neuroendocrine Disorders

Rare but life-threatening paraneoplastic syndromes can be triggered by squamous cell carcinoma. These syndromes are generated by the tumor's impact on distant organs or systems. Paraneoplastic syndromes that can occur alongside SCC include hypercalcemia, thromboembolism, or inflammatory reactions that impact the skin, joints, or nerves. The identification and management of paraneoplastic syndromes in SCC patients requires close monitoring of biochemical markers, imaging investigations, and consultation with experts such as endocrinologists or rheumatologists.

Effects on Well-Being

Squamous cell carcinoma is a serious cancer that, once diagnosed, can have a devastating effect on a patient's standard of living. Distress, both mental and physical, medication side effects, and alterations to one's way of life can all have an impact on one's state of health. To improve the quality of life and address the holistic requirements of patients with SCC, supportive care services are essential. These treatments include pain management, dietary assistance, psychiatric counseling, and rehabilitation.

Identifying SKUs and Kinds

There are many different kinds of squamous cell carcinoma, and they all look and feel different. Spindle cell carcinoma, adenosquamous carcinoma, basaloid squamous cell carcinoma, keratoacanthoma-like SCC, and verrucous carcinoma are some of the subtypes that can be found. For accurate prognostication and therapy planning, histological identification of these subgroups is crucial.

Squamous cell carcinoma (SCC) can present in a variety of ways depending on the location of the cancer, so it's important to assess the patient thoroughly, bring in experts from other fields to help, and put the patient first if you want the best possible outcome.

CHAPTER 4

ANALYSIS OF HEALTH STATUS

Health History and Physical Assessment

In a physical examination, the doctor will look for abnormalities on the skin, particularly in regions that are exposed to sunlight.

Sun exposure, prior skin malignancies, immunosuppression, and genetic predispositions are important risk factors to consider when reviewing the patient's medical history.

- It is important to note a family history of skin cancer, specifically squamous cell carcinoma (SCC).

Methods for Conducting Biopsies and Analysing Their Results

- A biopsy is a surgical procedure that includes removing a little piece of tissue to study it under a microscope.

The size and location of the lesion determine the technique used, which can be either a punch biopsy, a shave biopsy, or an excisional biopsy.

To confirm a diagnosis of SCC, histopathological investigation evaluates cell type, differentiation, invasion depth, and margins.

Radiological Imaging Techniques (X-ray, CT, MRI, PET-CT):

Bony invasion or metastases to the lungs might be seen on an X-ray.

MRI and CT scans can show the extent of invasion into bones and lymph nodes as well as any soft tissue involvement.

If you have a high-risk instance of SCC, PET-CT can help you find distant metastases.

Evaluation via Endoscopy:

Squamous cell carcinoma (SCC) in the throat, bladder, or esophagus can be evaluated via an endoscope.

To make informed treatment decisions, it is useful for assessing tumor size, invasion, and staging.

Investigations Conducted in a Lab (Weapons Analysis, Cancer Detectors)

Comprehensive blood counts (CBCs) and tests for kidney and liver function provide a snapshot of a patient's general health and the state of their organs.

Squamous cell carcinoma antigen (SCC-Ag) and other tumor markers may help track how well a patient is responding to treatment.

Genetic Analysis (NGS, PCR)

To guide targeted treatments, next-generation sequencing (NGS) and polymerase chain reaction (PCR) find genetic alterations linked to SCC.

For both prognosis and therapy response prediction, these tests are useful.

The Function of Liquid Biopsies:

-CTCs, cfDNA, and exosomes in blood and other body fluids are examined in liquid biopsies.

Non-invasive monitoring of SCC, treatment response assessment, and detection of minimum residual disease or recurrence are all possible with their help.

Standards for Radiological Staging

TNM staging is one set of criteria used in radiological staging, which evaluates tumor size, lymph node involvement, and distant metastases.

Treatment planning and prognosis are both aided by staging.

Diagnosis Through a Multidisciplinary Approach

The diagnosis of SCC frequently requires the participation of a multidisciplinary team that includes surgeons, radiologists, dermatologists, pathologists, and oncologists.

Working together, we can guarantee precise staging, diagnosis, and treatment programs tailored to each individual.

Diagnostic Obstacles and Difficulties

- One of the difficulties is telling SCC apart from other skin lesions such as basal cell carcinoma or keratoacanthoma.

- It may be difficult to diagnose invasive SCC variations or tumors with poor differentiation without the assistance of a specialist.

To effectively diagnose squamous cell carcinoma and provide early and suitable treatment customized to each patient's needs, it is essential to understand these elements.

CHAPTER 5

APPROACHES TO TREATMENT

Analysis of Margin and Resection Techniques in Surgery

When it comes to treating SCC, surgery is still essential. Mohs micrographic surgery and similar techniques allow for the accurate removal of tumors while minimizing injury to adjacent tissues. This is especially important for areas that are sensitive to aesthetics. For bigger tumors, it is typical to perform a wide local excision. To guarantee full removal, margin assessment is crucial, and permanent sections or frozen sections are frequently used either during or after surgery.

Techniques and Targeted Approaches in Radiation Therapy

In difficult or advanced instances, radiation can be a lifesaver. Methods such as intensity-modulated radiation treatment (IMRT) identify and destroy cancer cells with pinpoint accuracy while avoiding nearby healthy tissues. Small areas can be treated with large doses of radiation using stereotactic body radiation treatment (SBRT). To lessen the likelihood of radiation damage to healthy tissues, targeted methods such as proton therapy are being increasingly used.

Systemic treatments include molecularly targeted agents and chemotherapy

Radiation and chemotherapy work together to kill cancer cells that divide too quickly. Cisplatin and other platinum-based meds are the gold standard. Tumour biomarkers guide the use of molecularly targeted treatments like as EGFR inhibitors (e.g., cetuximab) or PD-1 inhibitors (e.g., pembrolizumab), which improve results while reducing side effects.

Immunotherapy New Approaches and Checkpoint Inhibitors

The immune system is strengthened to combat cancer with immunotherapy. Nivolumab and pembrolizumab are examples of checkpoint inhibitors that prevent cancer cells from escaping immune system responses by blocking the signals they employ. One innovative method that has shown encouraging outcomes in clinical studies is adoptive cell therapy, which uses modified T lymphocytes to target antigens specific to SCC.

Thermodynamic Phototherapy

In photodynamic treatment (PDT), light-activated photosensitizers are used to kill cancer cells. It helps with superficial SCCs, which are particularly common on the face and other cosmetically delicate places. PDT is appealing in some situations because it is non-invasive and leaves little scarring.

Electrochemotherapy is a treatment method.

By combining chemotherapy with electric pulses, electrochemotherapy increases the treatment efficacy by enhancing medication uptake by cancer cells. In cases where other therapies have failed or when surgery or radiation would be too invasive, it has shown to be an excellent option for treating SCCs.

Therapies Used in Combination

In cases of advanced SCC, the best results are achieved by combining various treatment techniques such as surgery, radiation, and chemotherapy. One example is the use of neoadjuvant chemotherapy before surgery, which reduces tumor size and makes resection easier. Improved local control and decreased recurrence rates are achieved with concurrent chemoradiation.

Management of Symptoms and Palliative Care

Patients with advanced SCC can expect their quality of life to be a primary focus of palliative treatment. It helps with things like physical discomfort, mental anguish, and exhaustion. All aspects of a patient's well-being, including their mental, emotional, and spiritual health, are taken into consideration by multidisciplinary teams.

Medicine as a Whole and Supplemental Treatments

In integrative medicine, complementary and alternative medicine (CAM) practices such as yoga, acupuncture, and herbal supplements are used in conjunction with mainstream therapy. These can help with treatment side effects, general health, and well-being while SCC is being treated.

Studies in Clinical Practice and Looking Ahead

Novel approaches to treating SCC, such as gene therapies, immunotherapies, and targeted medicines, are being investigated in clinical studies. They provide access to innovative treatments and provide important data for better management of SCC. Genetic profiling-based personalized medicine and cutting-edge immunotherapeutic approaches are two potential future avenues.

Better results, enhanced quality of life, and continuous improvements in treatment efficacy can be achieved by incorporating these patient-specific therapeutic modalities in SCC care.

CHAPTER 6

METHODS OF MANAGEMENT ORGAN SITE-BY-SITE

Squamous Cell Carcinoma of the Skin (CSCC)

- After melanoma, CSCC ranks high among skin cancers.

Radiation treatment for inoperable tumors, excisional surgery for localized lesions, or Mohs micrographic surgery for high-risk regions are all part of the management plan.

For tumors that pose a high risk of spreading, a sentinel lymph node biopsy could be an option to consider.

For superficial lesions or in situ disease, topical therapies such as imiquimod or 5-fluorouracil can be utilized.

Due to the danger of local recurrence and metastasis, it is necessary to have regular follow-ups.

Novel Squamous Cell Carcinoma of the Head and Neck (HNSCC)

Oral, pharyngeal, laryngeal, and paranasal sinus malignancies are all part of HNSCC.

- The patient, the stage, and the location all have a role in the management approach.

- Multiple specialists work together to determine the best course of treatment, which may involve surgery, radiation, chemotherapy, or a mix of these methods.

In some circumstances, methods for preserving organs, such as chemoradiation, may be employed.

For patients with severe or recurrent HNSCC, new treatments such as targeted therapy and immunotherapies are showing promise.

Carcinoma of the Oesophagus

Tobacco and alcohol consumption are frequently linked to esophageal squamous cell carcinoma.

- When the disease is in its early stages, surgical treatments such as esophagectomy or endoscopic resection are used for management.

Locally progressed or metastatic cancers are treated with chemo or radiation therapy.

Post-treatment monitoring and recurrence detection rely on endoscopic surveillance.

Carcinoma of the Lung Squamous Cells

30 percent of NSCLC cases are LSCC.

- Staging and molecular features dictate management.

- In the early stages of the disease, surgery is the main treatment option. However, in more advanced cases, chemotherapy, immunotherapy, or targeted therapy may be necessary.

- Treatment decisions are guided by molecular testing for mutations such as EGFR, ALK, and PD-L1 expression.

Carcinoma of the Cervical Squamous Cell

Squamous cell carcinomas account for the vast majority of cervical cancer cases.

Depending on the stage and extent of the disease, management may require a mix of radiation therapy, chemotherapy, and surgery.

Screening with HPV testing and Pap smears aids in the early detection and prevention of cervical cancer.

Cancer of the Anal Squamous Cell Line

- Linked to human papillomavirus infection, particularly in those living with HIV.

Surgery, irradiation, and chemotherapy are all part of the treatment, which can be administered in either a neoadjuvant or adjuvant context.

Colorectal surgeons, oncologists, and radiation oncologists must work together to treat anal cancer.

The Cancer of the Genital Squamous Cells

Vulva, vaginal, and penile SCCs are all part of this category.

Treatment options include radiation therapy, chemotherapy, and surgery, depending on the location and stage of the disease.

When it comes to vulvar and vaginal SCCs in particular, HPV vaccination is an important preventative measure.

One Kind of Oral Cancer OSCC

- Commonly linked to substances like alcohol and smoke, in addition to HPV infection.

Surgery, chemo, radiation, and other treatments may be considered while thinking about the patient's functional results and quality of life.

Patients receiving radiation therapy must undergo thorough dental evaluation and management to avoid problems.

Carcinoma of the Conjunctiva

Ocular cancer is uncommon but significant.

For localized disease, treatment options include surgical excision, cryotherapy, or topical chemotherapy.

Checking for recurrence or metastasis requires regular ophthalmologic follow-ups.

Sites Uncommon and Uncommon Presentations

- SCCs that appear in unusual places, such as the ear, scalp, or perianal area, fall under this category.

Treatment is based on standard operating procedures (SOPs) for surgery, radiation, and chemotherapy, adjusted according to the location and stage of the patient's cancer.

The key to a correct diagnosis and the best possible treatment is tight cooperation between doctors and pathologists.

The management strategy for squamous cell carcinoma always includes patient education, supportive care, and regular follow-ups. Each patient receives individualized, comprehensive care from multidisciplinary teams that include surgeons, oncologists, radiologists, pathologists, and others in the medical field.

CHAPTER 7

MONITORING AND FOLLOW-UP TREATMENT

Protocols for Post-Treatment Monitoring

It is critical to observe for symptoms of recurrence or problems after squamous cell carcinoma treatment. As part of these protocols, patients are usually required to undergo imaging scans, blood tests, and physical examinations. Stage and kind of cancer determine how often patients must return for follow-up consultations, which may be more frequent at the outset and gradually spaced out if all goes well.

As part of imaging surveillance, imaging tests such as computed tomography (CT), magnetic resonance imaging (MRI), and positron emission tomography (PET) can be utilized to identify the presence or progression of tumors. An individual's risk factors and cancer treatment history are the primary determinants of the imaging frequency and type.

Monitoring Biomarkers

Biomarkers are naturally occurring substances that can reveal whether cancer is present or how well a patient is responding to treatment. To detect early indications of recurrence or to evaluate the efficacy of treatment, it is possible to monitor particular biomarkers using blood tests or other means.

Cancer treatment records, possible side effects, and suggestions for follow-up care are all part of a survivor's care plan. They typically provide details on where to get emotional support, how to live a healthy lifestyle, and how to deal with any long-term negative effects.

Counselling and psychological support:

coping with a cancer diagnosis and its effects can be taxing on mental health. If a patient is struggling with anxiety, despair, or any other mental health issue, having access to psychological services such as counseling and support groups may be life-changing.

Cancer therapies, including radiation, chemotherapy, and surgery, can bring about a variety of side effects. Whether they appear suddenly or gradually, these side effects can be managed as part of follow-up treatment to enhance quality of life and general health.

The key to effective treatment is early detection of cancer recurrence, which is important for recurrence management. Patients are motivated to report any changes that may be cause for worry and are informed about possible symptoms to keep an eye out for. Depending on the individual instance, recurrent squamous cell carcinoma treatment options could involve immunotherapy, targeted therapy, radiation therapy, chemotherapy, or surgery.

Ongoing Management of Long-Term Effects and Complications

Certain cancer treatments may cause problems or side effects that last a long time. Lymphedema, nerve damage, hormone abnormalities, and subsequent malignancies are all possible complications. These possible issues can be better monitored and treated with regular follow-up treatment.

The Role of Lifestyle Changes

Changing to a healthier way of life can greatly improve health and well-being and lessen the likelihood of cancer returning. This involves taking care of one's health in many ways, such as eating right, exercising regularly, not smoking and not drinking too much, dealing with stress, and seeing a doctor often.

One of the most important ways to get patients involved in their healthcare is through patient education and empowerment programs that teach them about their illness, their treatment choices, and how to take care of themselves. Patients are better able to make educated decisions and take charge of their health when they have access to educational resources, counseling, and support from healthcare professionals.

When combined, these components form an all-encompassing strategy for monitoring and follow-up care for patients treated with squamous cell carcinoma. Healthcare teams can help patients get the best results and live better lives by addressing their physical, mental, and lifestyle problems.

CHAPTER 8

TAKING PRECAUTIONS AND MINIMISING DANGER

Ways to Prevent Sun Damage

1. **Sun Protection and UV Exposure Awareness:** Spread the word about how dangerous UV rays are and why everyone should wear sunscreen.

2. **Sunscreen Use:** Recommend that people frequently use broad-spectrum sunscreens (SPF 30 or greater) when going outside.

3. **Protective Clothing:** Suggest that people avoid burning their skin by wearing long-sleeved shirts, sunglasses, and hats with wide brims.

4. To minimize exposure to ultraviolet radiation, it is recommended to seek shade throughout the middle of the day, between 10 a.m. and 4 p.m.

5. Encourage both self-examination and frequent dermatologist appointments as a means of preventing skin cancer.

Programmes to Help People Quit Smoking

1. **Raise Awareness and Education:** Inform the public about the connection between smoking and SCC and encourage them to quit.

2. Counselling and behavioral therapies can assist smokers in kicking the habit and making positive lifestyle changes.

3. Make available nicotine replacement therapy (NRT) items like patches, gum, and lozenges so people can cope with the symptoms of nicotine withdrawal.

4. Facilitate online communities or support groups where people may talk to each other about their struggles and get encouragement while they try to quit.

Methods for Vaccination (e.g., Human papillomavirus)

To prevent HPV-related SCC, it is recommended that individuals, particularly teenagers and young adults, get vaccinated against high-risk strains of the human papillomavirus (HPV).

2. **Educational Campaigns:** Bring attention to the correlation between HPV infection and SCC, stressing the need for immunization to ward against the disease.

Precautions for the Workplace

1. to identify possible carcinogens and hazards in work contexts, it is important to conduct comprehensive risk assessments.

2. To minimize exposure to dangerous compounds, it is important to provide suitable protective equipment such as goggles, gloves, and masks.

3. **Education and Training:** Provide courses on safe work practices, such as how to handle dangerous materials and how to keep the workplace free of hazards.

Suggestions for Food and Nutrition

1. **Healthy Eating Habits:** The risk of cancer is lowered when people eat a balanced diet that is high in fruits, vegetables, whole grains, and lean proteins.

2. **Reducing Exposure to Carcinogenic Substances:** Suggest cutting back on alcoholic beverages, processed meats, and foods heavy in sugar and bad fats.

3. **Hydration:** Stress the significance of drinking enough water to maintain healthy skin and proper skin function.

Anti-Chemical Measures

1. When it comes to chemoprevention in high-risk patients, it's worth looking into topical treatments like retinoids and nonsteroidal anti-inflammatory medications (NSAIDs).

2. Encourage people to take part in clinical trials that study new chemopreventive drugs or ways to avoid SCC.

3. Risk assessment involves finding those who are more likely to develop SCC and could benefit from chemopreventive treatments, such as those who have a family history of the disease or a history of precancerous lesions.

Campaigns for Early Detection

1. **Screening Programmes:** Promote the need for routine SCC screenings, particularly for at-risk populations including those with fair skin or a family history of sunburn.

2. **Awareness Campaigns:** Spread the word about squamous cell carcinoma (SCC) symptoms

and signs to encourage people to see worrisome lesions quickly and get medical help.

3. **Provider Training:** Educate medical professionals on how to spot SCC in its early stages, so patients can get treatment sooner rather than later.

Mitigating Environmental Risk Factors

1. Environmental pollution and exposure to carcinogenic contaminants may play a role in the development of SCC; therefore, it is important to support measures that try to reduce pollution.

2. The purpose of UV index monitoring is to raise awareness about days with excessive UV exposure and to encourage people to take precautions by using UV index forecasts.

3. Promoting green areas, shade structures, and UV-protective components in public spaces should be a priority in urban development.

Screening and Genetic Counselling

1. People who have a history of SCC in their family or who are known to have a genetic predisposition to skin cancer should be offered genetic testing as well as counseling services.

2. To identify individuals at elevated risk of developing SCC, it is necessary to conduct detailed risk assessments based on hereditary variables.

3. Customise sun protection, screening, and lifestyle changes to each person's unique genetic risk profile as part of a comprehensive preventative program.

Programmes and Policies for Public Health

1. **Lawmaking:** Push for rules and laws that increase awareness of the need for sun protection in public settings, including schools and workplaces.

2. **Funding Support:** Raise money to support public health programs that aim to reduce the occurrence of SCC. These programs should include activities to educate the public, conduct research, and increase access to preventive services.

3. **Collaborative Efforts:** Encourage healthcare organizations, advocacy groups, government agencies, and community stakeholders to work together to adopt nationwide and local plans that prevent SCC.

In a comprehensive strategy to reduce the likelihood of squamous cell carcinoma, each of these factors—ranging from personal actions to public health policies and programs—is essential.

CHAPTER 9

ADVOCACY AND THE VIEWS OF PATIENTS

Stories of Patients' Journeys

A patient journey narrative is an effective tool for documenting the events surrounding a squamous cell carcinoma diagnosis, therapy, and beyond. These accounts give readers a glimpse into the patients' experiences by detailing the mental, physical, and emotional struggles they encountered. The effects of SCC on their everyday lives, important milestones, treatment choices, and supporting care are frequently highlighted. Storytelling about a patient's story may do wonders for spreading awareness, encouraging compassion, and uniting patients and carers.

Groups and Resources to Help

Squamous cell carcinoma patients greatly benefit from attending support groups where they can find understanding, helpful information, and a community of like-minded individuals. Healthcare providers, patient advocates, or non-profits frequently host these groups, which can meet in person or virtually. They provide a welcoming environment where people with SCC may talk about their experiences, get accurate information, and make connections with others who understand what it's like to live with the disease. Helplines, educational materials, and informational websites all play a role in providing patients and carers with the knowledge and assistance they need.

Groups that Speak Out for Causes

Squamous cell carcinoma advocacy groups fight for better healthcare policies and patient access to high-quality treatment by raising public knowledge of the disease and its effects, advocating for patient's rights, and funding research projects. To meet the needs of people with SCC and bring about good change, these groups work together with healthcare practitioners, researchers, legislators, and the community. Participation in clinical trials and other research projects, as well as educational programs and advocacy campaigns, financial aid, and other opportunities are common offerings.

Programmes for Peer Mentorship

Squamous cell carcinoma patients might find support from mentors who have been through it all through peer mentorship programs. Patients' resilience, decision-making capacity, and ability to traverse the healthcare system are all improved via these programs' facilitation of peer-to-peer support, counseling, and encouragement. By sharing their experiences with SCC, peer mentors encourage mentees and give them tools for resilience and self-sufficiency.

Resilience and Coping Mechanisms

Living with squamous cell carcinoma is challenging in every way; coping mechanisms are necessary for handling the mental, emotional, and practical challenges. Methods for cultivating awareness and acceptance of one's internal and external environments, as well as for managing symptoms of pain and stress, may be part of these plans. Resilience training is essential because it teaches patients to overcome obstacles, keep a positive attitude, and adjust to new circumstances as they face SCC.

Effects on Friends, Family, and Carers

Everyone involved in caring for a patient with squamous cell carcinoma feels its effects. As they help their loved ones through the diagnosis, treatment, and recovery processes, carers frequently face emotional distress, carer burden, financial difficulties, and changes to their way of life. As part of comprehensive care for SCC patients and their families, it is vital to recognize and address the needs of carers. This includes providing education, respite care, and support services to carers.

Taking Care of People's Mental and Emotional Health

Patients with squamous cell carcinoma must get comprehensive care that includes emotional and psychological assistance. During their journey with SCC, patients may go through a variety of emotions, including fear, worry, sadness, rage, loss, and uncertainty. Psychosocial assistance, counseling, and access to oncology-focused mental health specialists are crucial for meeting these needs. The emotional health and quality of life of SCC patients can be improved by the promotion of self-care, the provision of coping skills, and the encouragement of open communication.

Aptitude for Health Information Exchange and Literacy

A person's health literacy level is a measure of how well they can read, comprehend, and apply health information to their own healthcare decisions. Patients with squamous cell carcinoma might benefit from improved health literacy if they are given accurate, easily understandable information regarding their disease, treatment choices, possible adverse effects, self-care, and follow-up appointments. To promote shared decision-making, establish trust, and guarantee good care coordination, it is crucial to improve communication skills among patients, carers, and healthcare practitioners.

Encouraging Patients to Take Part in Decision-Making

Involving squamous cell carcinoma patients as active participants in their care journey is key to empowering them in decision-making. Respecting their beliefs, aspirations, and preferences entails giving them thorough information about their diagnosis, treatment options, risks, advantages, and possible outcomes. Better treatment adherence, patient satisfaction, and results for SCC patients are achieved by shared decision-making, which fosters autonomy, teamwork, and patient-centered care.

Helping More People Have Access to Health Care

It is critical to guarantee that all people impacted by squamous cell carcinoma, irrespective of their background, socioeconomic level, or region, have access to high-quality healthcare and health equity. This necessitates resolving challenges with healthcare accessibility, such as insufficient funding, inadequate transportation, language hurdles, cultural factors, and healthcare delivery inequalities. To improve health equality and outcomes for SCC patients, it is vital to advocate for policies that encourage equitable care, fund outreach programs, and collaborate with community stakeholders.

All of these things work together to make squamous cell carcinoma treatment more patient-centered by highlighting the significance of patients' and their families' agency, advocacy, support networks, and holistic care.

CHAPTER 10

A GLOBAL VIEW AND A LOOK AHEAD

The Worldwide Impact of Squamous Cell Carcinoma

One of the leading causes of cancer deaths worldwide is squamous cell carcinoma. While the skin is the most common site of infection, it can also manifest in other organs such as the cervix, esophagus, and lungs. Skin squamous cell carcinoma (SCC) is a prevalent kind of skin cancer that can vary in frequency depending on factors such as population demographics, sun exposure rates, and geographical location. To create efficient treatment and prevention plans, it is essential to comprehend this load.

Variations in Morbidity and Prognosis

The occurrence and survival rates of SCC vary greatly among populations and locales. Some of the factors that can impact these differences include cultural customs, financial status, education levels, and access to healthcare. Reducing these inequalities requires tackling social determinants of health, raising awareness, expanding screening programs, boosting access to excellent healthcare, and more.

Collaborations and Research on a Global Scale

Improving our knowledge of SCC relies heavily on international research and collaborations. Researchers, physicians, legislators, and patient advocates from all over the globe come together in collaborative projects to exchange information, resources, and best practices. The discovery of novel diagnostic tools, preventative measures, and therapeutic interventions is sped up by these partnerships.

New Approaches to Healthcare Delivery and Technology

The detection and treatment of SCC have been transformed by technological advancements. Minimally invasive surgical treatments, tailored medications, immunotherapy, targeted imaging, and molecular diagnostics have all contributed to better patient outcomes. Healthcare systems that include these technologies improve accuracy, productivity, and patient happiness.

Economic Analysis of Health Care and Interventions with Minimal Cost

When it comes to SCC, health economics is vital. Reducing financial burdens on patients and healthcare systems while optimizing healthcare resources and increasing outcomes are the goals of cost-effective therapies. Health technology evaluations, value-based care, and novel payment structures are some of the strategies that can help ensure that everyone has access to high-quality care in the future.

Personalized Treatments and Precision Medicine

Squamous cell carcinoma (SCC) treatment has been radically altered by precision medicine. Customizing treatments to each patient's unique genetic, molecular, and clinical traits is the essence of this approach. Treatment efficacy, side effect management, and patient outcomes are all improved by personalized approaches. Precision medicine plays an essential role in the management of SCC through biomarker-driven medicines and genetic profiling.

Problems with Putting Best Practices into Action

The implementation of best practices for SCC remains a difficulty, notwithstanding progress. Regulatory complexity, gaps in patient education, healthcare infrastructure inequities, and restricted access to innovative therapies are among these issues. Collaborations between various stakeholders changes to policies, and efforts to continuously enhance quality are all necessary to tackle these difficulties.

Healthcare Models Focused on Patients

When it comes to SCC, patient-centric healthcare models put the patient's wants, requirements, and values first. These methods emphasize psychological therapies, survivorship care planning, extensive support services, and collaborative decision-making. Improvements in treatment adherence, patient happiness, and general health can be achieved by involving patients as active participants in their healthcare.

Concerns Regarding Ethics in Cancer Care

To provide fair and compassionate cancer care, ethical issues must be carefully considered. Important considerations include cultural competency, end-of-life care, informed consent, privacy protection, and resource allocation. To help healthcare providers make ethical decisions that promote justice, autonomy, and dignity for patients with SCC, ethical frameworks are used.

Positive Movements and Encouragement

Research and treatment for SCC face obstacles, however, there are encouraging trends and progress. Early detection methods, combination treatments, immunotherapy, targeted medicines, and targeted therapeutics are revolutionizing patient outcomes. New developments in the treatment of SCC may be on the horizon thanks to ongoing clinical trials, the identification of biomarkers, and translational research.

Research, innovation, collaboration, equity, ethics, and patient-centered treatment are all essential components of a complete strategy to tackle the worldwide impact of squamous cell carcinoma. Patients with SCC have reason to be optimistic about the future because of developments in precision medicine, healthcare delivery methods, and technology.

www.ingramcontent.com/pod-product-compliance
Lightning Source LLC
Chambersburg PA
CBHW071839210526
45479CB00001B/209